Written by:
Olivia Rashwalb

Medically Reviewed by:
Gur Rashwalb, MD

A Systematic Review

Cover design by: Olivia Rashwalb

Abstract

Throughout history, society has viewed ADHD and ADHD-like behavior differently. Often, those without ADHD are ignorant to the disorder, and label individuals with ADHD as lazy, disorganized, and cognitively inferior to others. For the longest time, caregivers, instructors, and peers attributed hyperactive and inattentive behavior on the students' will to impede success. However, researchers found reasons for these behaviors. Due to the knowledge and strategies to support the needs of individuals with ADHD, individuals with ADHD have become more successful. In addition, for a long time, there has been many debates over ADHD: many debate ADHD medications; ADHD as the primary disorder or the comorbidity; alternative labels for ADHD; and ADHD's existence. However, those opposing ADHD's existence, excuse the symptoms as lack of responsibility. A neutral perspective recognizes ADHD as a real disorder, acknowledging its difficulties, and feeding it's creativity and recognizing that there is not just one way to treat the disorder, thus, motivating individuals with ADHD to succeed. There are many ways to treat ADHD, such as synthetic medication and external support (academically and socially). Others believe in controversial alternative labels and treatment methods for ADHD. Supporting ADHD will prevent the unfair stigma surrounding ADHD. This stigma lowers self esteem, and motivation to succeed.

Attention Deficit/ Hyperactivity Disorder

A Systematic Review

Olivia P. Roshwalb
Medically Reviewed by: Dr. Gur Roshwalb

Olivia P. Roshwalb
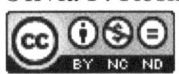
Attention Deficit/ Hyperactivity Disorder: A Systematic Review by Olivia P. Roshwalb is licensed under a Creative Commons Attribution-NonCommercial-NoDerivatives 4.0 International License.
ISBN-13: 978-1523378920
ISBN-10: 1523378921

To my friends and family for your constant encouragement. To my parents, Gur and Valerie Roshwalb, and my siblings, Arianne, Raphael, and Ariel Roshwalb, for giving me all your love and support. To my eighth grade social studies teacher, Mr. Coughlan, for inspiring me and assigning this essay. To everyone with ADHD-- YOU CAN DO IT. To Jessica Romano, and Jennifer Gutstein for providing me with your insight on ADHD.

Contents

Acknowledgements...i
Letter To Readers..ii
Introduction...2
Historical, Diagnostic, and Genetic Information...8
Ways to support and cope with ADHD.............23
Medication..30
Controversy of Indigo Children....................40
Conclusion..50

Acknowledgements

I thank Dr. Gur Roshwalb, M.D. for medically reviewing this manuscript. I would also like to express my infinite gratitude towards Ms. Jessica Romano, a learning specialist at Ethical Culture Fieldston School, and Ms. Jennifer Gutstein, LCSW-R, for sharing their understanding of ADHD with me throughout the advancement of this "investigation." I am also grateful to Mr. Joseph Coughlan of S.A.R. Academy, for assigning this paper. In addition, I must also thank my grandparents, Mamie, Papi, Saba and Savta, and my family, Maman, Papa, Arianne, Raphael, Ariel, Yael, Shay, Kelly and Guershon for constantly showing me your love and support. Lastly, I would like to separately thank, Dr. Esther Roshwalb, PhD., for inspiring me to take this paper into my own hands, and writing a professional article, just like you do, and Suzanne Susskind for showing me how to take my talents as a writer to help others, just like you do.

Letter to Readers

Dear Readers,
Let me introduce myself. My name is Olivia Roshwalb, and I am currently a highschool freshman with a passion for learning. I also have ADHD. When I was younger, before my diagnoses, I was often frustrated with myself, and teachers were often frustrated with me because I often lost focus and I didn't know what was going on in class. I had a really hard time organizing myself and my belongings, and I was "too independent." In fourth grade, we finally received a diagnosis, answers, to why I had so much trouble focusing and controlling my impulses. Throughout my years, I have dealt with my fair share of ignorant teachers, and students alike. I was put in a smaller group, and labeled as "stupid," when in reality I lost focus because I did not feel challenged. Since then, I have developed learning strategies, and now I am in very advanced classes. In eighth grade, my former social studies teacher, Mr. Joseph Coughlan, assigned a research paper on whatever we wanted. I decided to write my paper about ADHD, as I was already familiar with the subject. I took it upon myself to write a paper that looked like a formal journal article because this would be my outlet, my way to show the world that individuals with ADHD are smart too, and that everybodys' brains are wired differently. I wrote this paper to show myself that I can start a big project like this and finish it. I wrote this paper to inspire others with the disorder. Lastly, I wrote this

paper to show the world the importance of understanding ADHD. Whether you are reading this because you have ADHD, you are a parent with a child affected with ADHD, you are a clinician, or a teacher, or anything else, understanding ADHD at its fullest is crucial to helping yourself, your child, your patient, or your student.
Enjoy,
Olivia

Introduction

  Views about Attention Deficit Hyperactivity Disorder have changed over time in terms of how people view it. There is a lot of judgement of people who have attention difficulties that labels them as stupid, lazy, messy and cognitively inferior to others. In the past, parents, teachers and peers blamed hyper and inattentive behavior on willpower and a child's choice to impede success. While symptoms of ADHD can be attributed to not following through or procrastination, scientist and medical professionals have come to understand that there are reasons for these behaviors.

  Throughout history, ADHD-like behavior has been recognized but not understood as a disorder. Instead, symptoms of ADHD have been judged as bad behavior, or cognitive inferiority. In the 1950s, reasons to further investigate the symptoms of ADHD led to the discovery of the disorder, its impact on the individual and the impact on those close to the person. Further observation found patterns that became logical and demonstrated a reason to believe that ADHD is a struggle or a disorder, rather than the freewill to impede success.

 The recognition of ADHD as a disorder has led to a change in events. Better brain research and deeper understanding of the academic environment has brought children with ADHD into the spotlight, recognizing ways to understand them and help them learn. This has led to a variety of treatment options that include both behavioral techniques and medical interventions: schedules and structure, medical prescription, meditation, physical activity and talk therapy. There are also additional methods of treatment and understanding of ADHD that link energy and spiritualism, that although make sense for some, it is controversial in the scientific world. Due to the better brain research, societies' understanding of the disorder has changed greatly.

 ADHD requires further explanation because of people's ignorance to the reality of the disorder. People with ADHD are misunderstood and therefore, are not treated equally. ADHD, otherwise known as Attention Deficit Hyperactivity Disorder, is described in the DSM-V as "a persistent pattern of inattention and/or hyperactivity-impulsivity that interferes with development, has symptoms presenting in two or more settings (e.g. at home, school, or work), and negatively impacts directly on social, academic or occupational functioning". Looking back in time, in 1775, Melchior Adam Weikard declared ADHD as superficial behavior, without the ability to do anything in depth. He treated the symptoms with sensory deprivation: darkness, reducing stimulation, and then integrating sports such as gymnastics and horseback riding.[1] Weikard discovered the tropical Cinchona plant that appeared to have acted as the first pre-modern stimulant.[2] Later in the 18th Century, Sir Alexander Crichton declared ADHD as the inability to attend and described individuals as easily agitated.[3] In 1902, Sir George Frederic Still, the father of pediatrics, described ADHD as "dependent on three

---

[1] Barkley, RA; Peters, H (November 2012). "The earliest reference to ADHD in the medical literature? Melchior Adam Weikard's description in 1775 of attention deficit (Mangel der Aufmerksamkeit, Attentio Volubilis)". *J Atten Disord* **16** (8): 623–30. doi:10.1177/1087054711432309. PMID 22323122.
[2] "Tropical Plant Database Entry For: Quinine Bark (Cinchona)." *Tropical Plant Database Entry For: Quinine Bark (Cinchona).* N.p., n.d. Web. 19 Apr. 2015. <http://www.rain-tree.com/quinine.htm#.VTO1xmT710A>.
[3] Crichton, Alexander (1798). *An Inquiry Into the Nature and Origin of Mental Derangement: Comprehending a Concise System of the Physiology and Pathology of the Human Mind. And a History of the Passions and Their Effects*1. T. Cadell, Junior, and W. Davies.

factors, a cognitive relation to environment, moral consciousness and volition." [4] Children were described as very smart, yet morally compromised. Later, in 1954, "Ritalin," a methylphenidate used for fatigue and other psychological reasons, was introduced and successfully used for treating ADHD. This was a turning point for people with ADHD-like symptoms (ADHD was not yet recognized by the American Psychiatric Association) because the medication helped individuals control impulses that they were not able to control on their own. This led researchers to believe that ADHD-like symptoms were not a personality choice, rather, they were connected physiologically. This new breakthrough changed the lives of individuals with ADHD, forever. In 1968, the American Psychiatric Association recognized ADHD as a neurodevelopmental disorder and put it in the DSM (Diagnostic and Statistical Manual of Mental Disorders) II. Since 1968, there have been major changes in the way that the

---

[4] Lange, Klaus W., Susanne Reichl, Katharina M. Lange, Lara Tucha, and Oliver Tucha. "The History of Attention Deficit Hyperactivity Disorder." *Attention Deficit and Hyperactivity Disorders*. Springer Vienna, n.d. Web. 20 Mar. 2015.

psychiatric world has viewed ADHD.[5] This change in view has led to the greater understanding of ADHD.

With proper understanding and strategies to support the needs of individuals with ADHD, the success rate of people diagnosed with ADHD increased because society has recognized the disorder and tolerated resources to be implemented. There are many arguments to support and oppose the concept that ADHD as a true disorder that should be recognized. Those who support ADHD agree that allowing individuals to be who they are and providing extra time for tests and other support, is fair and equal. Individuals who oppose the reality of ADHD, often excuse the disorder as bad behavior, and lack of responsibility. However, a neutral perspective says that there are two sides of ADHD and not just one remedy. Recognizing ADHD as a real disorder and also accepting its challenges and embracing its creativity will motivate individuals to succeed.

ADHD should be noticed and supported instead of

---

[5] "ADHD: The Diagnostic Criteria." *PBS*. PBS, n.d. Web. 12 Apr. 2015.
<http://www.pbs.org/wgbh/pages/frontline/shows/medicating/adhd/diagnostic.html>.

labeling a child as cognitively inferior. The impact of labeling is destructive to self-esteem and being productive, which alters the outcome of one's life.

Historical, Diagnostic, and Genetic Information

ADHD has a long history that dates back as early as 493 BCE, during the time of Hippocrates. Before the world began to understand the disorder and neurodevelopment, people described difficulties with attention and hyperactivity in correlation with earthly elements. Hippocrates first described symptoms of what seems to be ADHD as an imbalance of fire over water, which made the person more fierce and hyperactive. Hippocrates treated this imbalance with dietary support: barley instead of wheat; fish instead of meat; water drinks instead of fruit drinks. Even in the early days of written history, ADHD-like behavior was acknowledged by an imbalance of impulses and behavior. These symptoms were treated with food to try and change the behavior of patients with ADHD-like symptoms.

In 1775, the earliest reference in medical literature, was written by Melchior Adam Weikard. He was interested in attention difficulties. Weikard believed that ADHD-like symptoms and behavior problems were attributed to the lack of structure in the home; blaming parents for their children's poor behavior. This was different from Hippocrates who clearly recognized the need to help the individual who was affected by these symptoms, as opposed to Weikard, who put the responsibility in the hands of the parents and dismissed the individual's needs. Weikard's remedy for these children were: physical activity such as horseback riding; sour milk; and in some cases, isolation to reduce outside stimuli. He also was the first to attempt a pre-modern stimulant from the Cinchona plant to calm these children down.

    The next advance in ADHD development was made by the father of pediatrics, George Frederic Still in 1902. Still focused on forty three children who were inattentive and hyperactive. These children had a short attention span and were often very impulsive, and were described as immoral, yet intelligent. This was the first documented statement describing the children as immoral. Still described the children with having difficulty at school academically and behaviorally, as well as socially. Frederic Still put forth a theory that there was a biological predisposition to this behavior. This development in research for ADHD helped the discovery of "Hyperactive Child Syndrome."

In 1937, Dr. Charles Bradley, administered benzedrine to a group of thirty misbehaved children, trying to subdue their headaches. He noticed that these children were more motivated academically, and around half these children were calmer, more obedient, and flexible. He noted, "The most striking change in behavior occurred in the school activities of many of these patients. There appeared a definite 'drive' to accomplish as much as possible. Fifteen of the thirty children responded to Benzedrine by becoming distinctly subdued in their emotional responses. Clinically in all cases, this was an improvement from the social viewpoint."[6] Unlike Sir Adam Weikard's herbal Cinchona treatment, Benzedrine was the first synthetic treatment for behavior disorders. Although this drug went unnoticed for about twenty five years, later benzedrine became a forerunner in treating ADHD with stimulants.

Since the early 1900s, before the Diagnostic and Statistical Manual for Mental Disorders (DSM), many researchers were interested in the causes of

---

[6] Strohl, Madeleine P. "Bradley's Benzedrine Studies on Children with Behavioral Disorders." *The Yale Journal of Biology and Medicine*. YJBM, n.d. Web. 28 May 2015.

behavioral and attention deficits. The encephalitis epidemic of 1917-1928 left many victims around the world with ADHD-like behavior; these symptoms included attention issues, hyperactivity, impulsivity and in some cases social detachment. In 1935, Dr. Kenneth E. Appel, and Earl D. Bond described postencephalitic children as "disobedient, untrainable at home or school," "inordinately restless," and strucken with "distractibility." In 1932, Franz Kramer, and Hans Pollow, described a precursor to ADHD, known then as "Hyperkinetic Disease of Infancy." This disease was characterized by extreme inattention, hyperactivity, and impulsivity.[7] Their method of treatment did not last long because of Thorazine's many hyper-intense side effects.[8] [9] This

---

[7] NEUMÄRKER, KLAUS-JÜRGEN. "The Kramer-Pollnow Syndrome: A Contribution on the Life and Work of Franz Kramer and Hans Pollnow." N.p., 2005. Web. Apr.-May 2015. <http%3A%2F%2Fwww.tara.tcd.ie%2Fbitstream%2Fhandle%2F2262%2F51558%2FPEER_stage2_10.1177%25252F0957154X05054708.pdf%3Fsequence%3D1%26isAllowed

[8] Some of the less serious side effects of Thorazine are dizziness, insomnia, anxiety, fatigue, weight gain, and constipation, however, some of the more serious side effect are nausea, seizures, tremors, rapid breathing, and flu-like symptoms.

[9] Thorazine (Chlorpromazine) Patient Information: Side Effects and Drug Images at RxList." *RxList*. N.p., n.d. Web.

early research lead to the modern understanding of ADHD. Despite the evidence that inattention and hyperactivity negatively affected some children, the first edition of the DSM did not mention attention or hyperactivity disorders, however the second edition of the DSM, the DSM II, recognized the impact of hyperactivity in some children. Hyperkinetic Reaction of Childhood was "overactivity, restlessness, distractibility, and short attention span, especially in young children; the behavior usually diminishes in adolescence."[10] The DSM-III recognized ADHD as Attention Deficit Disorder with and without hyperactivity. The DSM-III-R changed this to Attention Deficit Hyperactivity Disorder, however there were no subtypes because researchers were unable to find any indication that suggested otherwise. Unlike the DSM-III-R, the DSM-IV recognized different manifestations of the disorder; there were three subtypes of ADHD. The first subtype

---

16 May 2015.
<http://www.rxlist.com/thorazine-drug/patient-images-side-effects.htm
[10] Conrad, Peter. "The Medicalization of Society." *Google Books*. The Johns Hopkins University Press, 2007. Web. 16 May 2015.

was "ADHD-predominately inattentive type;" these children were very inattentive however they did not display excessive hyperactivity. The second subtype was "ADHD-predominantly hyperactive-impulsive type;" these children were not inattentive however they were extremely hyperactive. Other children displayed both excessive inattention and hyperactive-impulsive behavior, so they were placed under "ADHD – Combined Type." [11] Although the main criteria for ADHD is the same in the DSM-IV and the DSM-V, the DSM-V recognizes the co-occurrence of ADHD and Autism Spectrum Disorder, and the DSM-V provides examples to some of the criteria in order to aid in the diagnostic process of ADHD. Throughout the history of the DSM, major improvements have been made in the recognition of the disorder.

 The DSM-V lists the most recent diagnostic criteria for inattention and hyperactivity-impulsivity. The DSM-V states that ADHD is "a persistent pattern of inattention and/or hyperactivity-impulsivity that

---

[11] Bennett, Victoria. "ADD with Hyperactivity to ADHD Subtypes." *History of ADHD*. Wordpress, n.d. Web. 16 May 2015.
<http://adhdhistory.umwblogs.org/add-with-hyperactivity-to-adhd/>.

interferes with functioning or development." Symptoms of inattention include: lack of or paying too much attention to small details, inattention during tedious activities (an uninteresting class), often appears to be inattentive when directly spoken to (appears to be in "lala land"), unreliable (often fails to complete school work, chores, or other tasks), impairments in executive functioning (disorganized, loses important items (homework, keys, wallets...), difficulty organizing details in paragraphs, difficulty handing things in on time), and is easily distracted by irrelevant or external stimuli. Symptoms of hyperactivity include: fidgeting, foot or hand tapping, squirming, leaves seat when inappropriate (possibly during class, a meeting or another setting where staying seated it expected), riotous behavior ("often runs about or climbs in situations where it is inappropriate"), difficulty participating in recreational interests calmly, often behaves as if "driven by a motor," "talks excessively," and has difficulty waiting turn (impatient, difficulty waiting on line, interrupts others, finishes sentences, and answers questions before they are finished). Children who are six or older must exhibit at least six symptoms per criteria for at least six months, however, adults who are at least seventeen must exhibit at least five symptoms per criteria for at least six months, and symptoms must have been present prior to age twelve. In addition, clinicians should specify the severity of the disorder and if the disorder is in partial remission, meaning that the full criteria has been met however the symptoms have not been present for at least six months.[12] Recognizing the symptoms of ADHD is important because individuals with ADHD need the proper support, and their symptoms need to be managed and not pathologized.

    Many symptoms of ADHD are attributed to an imbalance of neurotransmitters and other hormones.[13] Those with Predominantly Inattentive

---

[12] Swedo, Susan E., M.D., Chair, Gillian Baird, M.A., M.B., B.Chir., Text Coordinator, Edwin H. Cook Jr., M.D., Francesca G. Happé, Ph.D., James C. Harris, M.D., Walter E. Kaufmann, M.D., Bryan H. King, M.D., Catherine E. Lord, Ph.D., Joseph Piven, M.D., Sally J. Rogers, Ph.D., Sarah J. Spence, M.D., Ph.D., Fred Volkmar, M.D., Amy M. Wetherby, Ph.D., and Harry H. Wright, M.D. "Neurodevelopmental Disorders." *Diagnostic and Statistical Manual of Mental Disorders: DSM-5.* 5th ed. Vol. I. Washington, D.C.: American Psychiatric Association, 2013. 59-65. Print. DSM.

[13] Neurotransmitters are hormones (chemicals) that transfer signals from one neuron (brain cell) to another neuron. This essay focuses on norepinephrine, dopamine, choline and serotonin.

type have mutations in the SLC6A2[14] gene, the norepinephrine transporter gene. Norepinephrine, a stress hormone, affects the parts of the brain dealing with attention and response;[15] it often works with epinephrine.[16] Those with Predominantly Hyperactive type of ADHD, have mutations to the DAT1[17] gene, the dopamine transporter gene. Dopamine is a neurotransmitter that helps manage things that relates to ADHD such as motor control, motivation, reward, sexual arousal and cognition.[18] Those with a combined presentation, have mutations in their

---

[14] Thakur, G.A., S.M. Sengupta, Z. Choudhry, and R. Joober. "Comprehensive Phenotype/genotype Analyses of the Norepinephrine Transporter Gene (SLC6A2) in ADHD: Relation to Maternal Smoking during Pregnancy." *National Center for Biotechnology Information*. U.S. National Library of Medicine, 20 Nov. 2012. Web. 27 May 2015.
[15] amygdala, cingulate gyrus, cingulum, hippocampus, hypothalamus, neocortex, spinal cord, striatum and thalamus
[16] Anonymous. "Norepinephrine." *SpringerReference* (2011): n. pag. *Rice*. Rice University. Web. 27 May 2015.
[17] *Genome Maps*. N.p., n.d. Web. 27 May 2015. <http://genomemaps.org/>.
[18] Jaber, M., S.W. Robinson, C. Missale, and M.G. Caron. "Dopamine Receptors and Brain Function." *National Center for Biotechnology Information*. U.S. National Library of Medicine, n.d. Web. 27 May 2015.

SLC5A7 gene,[19] the choline transporter gene. Choline, a Vitamin-B-like[20] neurotransmitter, prevents memory loss, and anxiety among other things, which may be the reason why individuals with ADHD need to be told things numerous times, and why they may experience mild anxiety. In addition to the neurotransmitters that affect learning, lack of serotonin (5HTTLPR gene)[21] causes impulsivity and aggression in ADHD.[22] In addition to genetic mutations in neurotransmitter transporter genes, there are other genetic factors associated with ADHD as well. Although there are a handful of genes that may be responsible for ADHD,[23] researchers believe that the genes mainly responsible are: Neurofibromin (NF1), and Latrophilin (LPHN3).[24] Neurofibromin

---

[19] *Genome Maps*. N.p., n.d. Web. 27 May 2015. <http://genomemaps.org/>.
[20] Aids in the synthesise of energy from food intake.
[21] *Genome Maps*. N.p., n.d. Web. 27 May 2015. <http://genomemaps.org/>.
[22] Zhang, Liuyan, Suhua Chang, Zhao Li, Kunlin Zhang, Yang Du, Jurg Ott, and Jing Wang. "ADHDgene: A Genetic Database for Attention Deficit Hyperactivity Disorder." *Nucleic Acids Research*. Oxford University Press, n.d. Web. 27 May 2015.
[23] Collingwood, Jane. "The Genetics of ADHD." *Psych Central*. N.p., n.d. Web. 27 May 2015.
[24] Van Der Voet, M., B. Harich, B. Franke, and A. Schenck. "ADHD-associated Dopamine Transporter, Latrophilin and

manages cognition, visual learning, and plays a major role in neurological cell development. Latrophilin "causes a reduction and misplacement of dopamine-positive neurons in the ventral diencephalon[25] and a hyperactive/impulsive motor phenotype."[26] [27] Although Genetics are not the only risk factors for ADHD, they play an important role in its etiology.

Like many neurodevelopmental disorders, other mental disorders co-occur and need to be managed; these co-occurring disorders are known as comorbidities. Common general comorbidities of ADHD are but not limited to: Conduct Disorders,

---

Neurofibromin Share a Dopamine-related Locomotor Signature in Drosophila." *National Center for Biotechnology Information*. U.S. National Library of Medicine, n.d. Web. 27 May 2015.

[25] The Thalamus (manages vision, auditory processing, sleeping, and touch) and Hypothalamus (secretes hormones) make up the Diencephalon.

[26] The physical and biological traits of an organism that is bound by the communication of its genetic nature and it's surroundings.

[27] Lange, M., W. Norton, M. Coolen, M. Chaminade, S. Merker, F. Proft, A. Shmitt, P. Vernier, K.P. Lesch, and L. Bally-Cuif. "The ADHD-susceptibility Gene Lphn3.1 Modulates Dopaminergic Neuron Formation and Locomotor Activity during Zebrafish Development."*National Center for Biotechnology Information*. U.S. National Library of Medicine, n.d. Web. 27 May 2015.

Depression and Anxiety disorders, Mood and Bipolar disorders, and any specific Learning Disorder.[28] Dr. Stephen Faraone, an expert in the comorbidities of ADHD, explains that because so many individuals with ADHD have other comorbidities, there is a debate as to whether in most cases ADHD is the primary disorder with other comorbidities, or a comorbidity to another disorder. "The nosological system advocated in the DSM is a hierarchical one. That is, in the presence of two or more diagnoses, one should be considered primary and account for many of the symptoms observed in the secondary syndrome. There is mounting evidence, however, that many conditions exist concurrently with ADHD, and each modify the overall clinical presentation and treatment response. These comorbid conditions should be considered simultaneously in order to broaden our understanding and maximize treatment".[29]

---

[28] Austin, Margaret, PH.D, Natalie S. Reiss, PH.D, and Laura Burgdorf, PH.D. "ADHD Comorbidity." *Mental Help.* CenterSite, LLC, 5 Nov. 2007. Web. 16 May 2015. <https%3A%2F%2Fwww.mentalhelp.net%2Farticles%2Fadhd-comorbidity%2F>.

[29] "ADHD and Comorbidity." *Medscape Medical Student.* Medscape, LLC, n.d. Web. <http%3A%2F%2Fwww.medscape.org%2Fviewarticle%2F418740>.

Attention Deficit Hyperactivity Disorder | Olivia Roshwalb

In November 2007, 21%-60% of children with ADHD showed symptoms of Oppositional Defiance Disorder (ODD), a conduct disorder; ODD is characterized by defiant and aggressive behavior towards authority figures. Researchers believe that children with ADHD develop ODD because of parental, and other disciplinarian figures frustration towards hyperactive and inattentive behavior.[30] In addition to ODD, in January of 2014, 22% of individuals with ADHD also experienced minor depression.[31] Depression may be associated with natural consequence of having ADHD; individuals with the disorder often view their daily environment as inconsistent (associated with impairments in executive functioning),[32] they may experience

---

[30] Turgay, Atilla, and Rubaba Ansari. "Major Depression with ADHD: In Children and Adolescents." *Psychiatry (Edgmont)*. Matrix Medical Communications, n.d. Web. 16 May 2015. <http://www.ncbi.nlm.nih.gov/pmc/articles/PMC2990565/>.
[31] "Statistical Prevalence of ADHD." *Statistical Prevalence of ADHD*. N.p., n.d. Web. 16 May 2015. <http://help4adhd.org/en/about/statistics#General>.
[32] Morin, Amanda. "Understanding Your Child's Trouble With Organization and Time Management." *Understood*. UNDERSTOOD.ORG USA LLC, n.d. Web. 17 May 2015. <https%3A%2F%2Fwww.understood.org%2Fen%2Flearning-attention-issues%2Fchild-learning-disabilities%2Forganiza

constant peer rejection (due to the "annoying" hyperactive behavior)[33], and they may view school as a place for failure. Furthermore, in January 2014, 15% of individuals with ADHD suffered from Generalized Anxiety Disorder. These individuals may experience "unpredictable mood swings (i.e., someone is happy one minute and miserable the next), excessive irritability, frequent angry outbursts, a noticeable lack of energy at times, and low self-esteem (particularly when individuals with ADHD start to recognize their own limitations in comparison to others). Other symptoms include frequent school absenteeism, somatic (physical) complaints, unwillingness to attempt new tasks, and a sense of resignation regarding their decreased ability to perform various tasks."[34] These children may also

---

tion-issues%2Funderstanding-your-childs-trouble-with-organization-and-time-management>.
[33] Morin, Amanda. "Understanding ADHD." *Understood.* UNDERSTOOD.ORG USA LLC, n.d. Web. <https%3A%2F%2Fwww.understood.org%2Fen%2Flearning-attention-issues%2Fchild-learning-disabilities%2Fadd-adhd%2Funderstanding-adhd%23item4>.
[34] Austin, Margaret, PH.D, Natalie S. Reiss, PH.D, and Laura Burgdorf, PH.D. "ADHD Comorbidity." *Mental Help.* CenterSite, LLC, 5 Nov. 2007. Web. 16 May 2015. <https%3A%2F%2Fwww.mentalhelp.net%2Farticles%2Fadhd-comorbidity%2F>.

experience lack of impetus due to the false realization that their actions do not make a difference in the lives of themselves or others. Moreover, in 2007, 10%-22% of children with ADHD also had Bipolar Disorder (57%-98% of individuals with Bipolar Disorder also have ADHD). As a matter of fact, many symptoms of ADHD and Bipolar Disorder such as inattention, hyperactivity-impulsivity, agitation, and bad sleeping patterns (hyperactive individuals tend to "keep going" for a very long time) overlap.[35] Additionally, 50% of children with ADHD also have learning disorders such as Dyslexia. In 2011, 25% of children with ADHD had Dyslexia and 15%-40% of children with Dyslexia also had ADHD.[36] Comorbidities of ADHD should be managed as they co-occur, in order to prevent further disruptions in the daily lives of individuals with ADHD.

---

[35] Faraone, Stephen V., PhD, and Arun R. Kunwar, MD. "ADHD in Children With Comorbid Conditions: ADHD and Bipolar Disorder." *Medscape Medical Student*. Medscape Psychiatry, 2007. Web. 17 May 2015.
[36] Vann, Madeline, MPH. "Is It ADHD or Dyslexia – or Both?" *EverydayHealth.com*. Ed. Pat F. Bass III. Everyday Health Media, LLC, 2015. Web. 17 May 2015.

Ways to support and cope with ADHD

When managing ADHD, teachers, parents, clinicians and the individual with ADHD should focus on treating the disorder academically, socially and in the home. When managing ADHD at school, teachers should keep in mind their students' ages, intelligent quotients (IQ), academic strengths and weaknesses, learning and organization style, severity and type of the disorder, and coping with the inattentive and hyperactive behavior. Teachers, parents and students with the disorder have the responsibility of enforcing appropriate accommodations. In addition to managing ADHD academically, when managing the disorder in social settings, clinicians should discuss the social impact of the disorder, establishing relationships, and self-awareness of the disorder. Lastly, when managing the disorder at home, parents, and clinicians should discuss ways to control the hyperactivity and impulsivity, and strategies to help their child organize their chores, and tasks. If ADHD is not managed at school, in social settings, and the home, the severe impact may destroy the individual's grounding. The recognition of ADHD has changed how people think and react towards the disorder. Greater understanding of ADHD positively impacts the overall course of treatment.

Teachers are semi-responsible for managing ADHD in the classroom. When looking at treating hyperactivity in the classroom, teachers must look at age and developmental level of their students with ADHD; for younger students, some experts recommend taping a square on the child's desk where the child can move freely[37] and, older students should be allowed to go for a short walk around the building every so often. Despite most people's' beliefs about students with ADHD, many students with ADHD have average and above average scores on IQ (intelligent quotient) testing; in the general population in 2000-2005, 15.86% of test takers score above average[38], however 27% of test takers with ADHD score above average[39], suggesting that these students

---

[37] "End Impulsive Behavior | 40 Best Accommodations for Your ADHD Child." *ADDitude Magazine*. New Hope Media LLC, n.d. Web. 20 May 2015.

[38] "IQ Scores - Average IQ Score at IQ Test Center." *IQ Scores - Average IQ Score at IQ Test Center*. N.p., n.d. Web. 20 May 2015.

[39] Kaplan, Bonnie J., Susan G. Crawford, Deborah M. Dewey, and Geoff C. Fisher. "The IQs of Children with

with ADHD may be cognitively superior to at least 84.14% of their peers. Likewise, teachers should also pay attention to their students' academic strengths and weaknesses. Students with ADHD become inattentive when board. However, they may become hyper-attentive when interested. Teachers should do things to attract the student's attention especially during classes where these students are less interested. Experts recommend that teachers have a "secret code" with the students; this "code" can include tapping students on the shoulder when they become inattentive,[40] and different signals indicating that the following is important (for example clapping before instructions).[41] Teachers should also repeat the directions and have at least three other students in the classroom repeat the directions so the student with ADHD has multiple opportunities to internalize the directions. In addition to this, teachers may also recommend learning specialists such as organization

---

ADHD Are Normally Distributed." Thesis. 2000. *Journal of Learning Disabilities* Volume 33 (2000): 425-32. Print.
[40] "Focus at School | 40 Best Accommodations for Your ADHD Child."*ADDitude Magazine.* N.p., n.d. Web. 20 May 2015.
[41] "Focus at School | 40 Best Accommodations for Your ADHD Child."*ADDitude Magazine.* N.p., n.d. Web. 20 May 2015.

tutors to help with school work and time management. Experts also recommend giving students with ADHD less work and more time to do the assignment so the student has a chance[42] to complete their assignment with their full potential. Similarly, students with ADHD are protected by the Individuals with Disabilities Education Act (IDEA) and are given extra time for tests.[43] Unfortunately, many students without the disorder and teachers alike, believe that these accommodations are unfair, however, ADHD is a disorder, and like all disorders and disabilities, accommodations must be made. That is to say, someone in a wheelchair is allowed privileged access to an elevator that nobody else is allowed to use because this person is unable to move up and down the staircase. Others in the building may complain that this is unjust because their lives would be much easier if they did not have to climb the stairs every day. By the same token, students with learning disabilities, such as ADHD, are provided extra time because they are unable to complete the test in the

---

[42] Gutstein, J. (2015, May 20th). Personal interview.
[43] United States of America. U.S. Department of Education. *Individuals with Disabilities Education Act Amendments of 1997*. N.p.: n.p., n.d. Web. 20 May 2015. <https://www2.ed.gov/policy/speced/leg/idea/idea.pdf>.

given time (due to inattention, distractibility, disorganization, hyperactivity, etcetera); in this case, ADHD is the wheelchair, and the extra time for tests is the elevator, the main difference is that people can see the wheelchair and its impact on the individual who needs it, but usually are unable to see the impacts of ADHD on the individual with the disorder. The external support and accommodations for students with ADHD positively affects their academic performance as well as their self-esteem.

    In addition to managing ADHD at school, some individuals with the disorder seek social counselling as well via Behavioral and/or Talk Therapies, and Social Skills Therapy. Aside from discussing personal feelings, clinicians discuss being self-aware of inattentive and hyperactive behavior along with social skills and establishing relationships. Clinicians and their patients may rehearse common conversations, confronting a bully, and making new friends. They may also discuss the social norm.[44] Learning social skills is important for some children with ADHD because friends build up confidence.

---

[44] Gutstein, J. (2015, May 20th) Personal interview.

Furthermore, the families of these individuals also work on managing ADHD in the home because for the most part, parents decide their child's treatment route. For instance, teachers and clinicians may suggest medication, however, the parents ultimately decide whether their child should be placed on medication. When assigning weekly chores, parents should use charts, and when giving smaller tasks, break up the tasks and assign them in smaller fragments; for example, instead of asking the child with ADHD to put plates, cups, and napkins on the table, rather the parents should ask their child to put plates on the table, when their child is done putting the plates on the table, then ask to set the cups, and when the child is finished putting the cups on the table, then ask to place the napkins on the table. In addition to this, parents should keep in mind that their child with ADHD often becomes sidetracked while doing tasks so constant reminders to stay on task may be necessary. Furthermore, experts recommend a reward system where parents constantly remind their children how to behave and when their children behave, rewards are given.[45] Managing ADHD

---

[45] Romano, J. (2015, May 21th) Personal interview.

appropriately in the home is important because this will provide the child with ADHD basic resources that they need to manage ADHD by themselves without the constant support.

Medication

Although medication does not work for everybody, it is a common treatment for ADHD. Common medication types include psychostimulants, and non-stimulants, however they are sometimes given together. When taking medication, individuals with ADHD, or their parents should understand how they work and their side effects. Similarly, the doctor prescribing the medication should be aware of the other medications that their patients are taking because certain medications will react negatively with the stimulant. Furthermore, medication is not a cure, and it is used to manage symptoms. Also, doctors like to try multiple medications and doses in order to find the perfect medication. When taking medication, understanding the expected effects is important as this helps tailor therapy to the individual.

Psychostimulants are the most common medication used to treat ADHD. There are many types of psychostimulants such as methylphenidate, dexmethylphenidate, amphetamine and dextroamphetamine. Concerta and Ritalin are both methylphenidates, however Ritalin works short term while Concerta works longer. Methylphenidates work by blocking the dopamine transporters,[46] hence the dopamine builds up in the synapse.[47] [48] In addition to Concerta and Ritalin, Focalin, a dexmethylphenidate is a stronger version of methylphenidate; these both increase the amount of dopamine.[49] Adderall is a combination of amphetamine and dextroamphetamine. Like the drugs listed above, these drugs also increase the dopamine levels in the brain, however, methylphenidate metabolizes faster. Although these are all similar stimulants, they each work a differently to increase the brain's dopamine levels.

  Stimulants are used to increase dopamine levels, however, individuals with the disorder may react to each psychostimulant differently. Recognizing the side effects of each psychostimulant is important because psychostimulant medication is usually determined by which side effects the patient

---

[46] The dopamine transporter manages the distribution of dopamine into neurons.
[47] In this case, a synapse is a network that allows a neuron to pass chemical signals to another neuron.
[48] Gottlieb, Scott. "Methylphenidate Works by Increasing Dopamine Levels."*BMJ : British Medical Journal.* BMJ, n.d. Web. 27 May 2015.
[49] "Dexmethylphenidate (Oral Route)." *Mayoclinic.org.* Thomson Healthcare Inc, n.d. Web. 27 May 2015.

can tolerate. Some less serious side effects of methylphenidate are nausea, loss of appetite, stomach pain, weight loss, vomiting, vision problems, dizziness, anxiousness, and insomnia, however some more serious and possibly lethal side effects are: allergic reaction, fever, arrhythmias, severe blistering, hallucinations, and dangerously high blood pressure; some individuals with heart conditions have suddenly died when taking methylphenidate.[50] The side effects of dexmethylphenidate are very similar to those of methylphenidate, however, dexmethylphenidate may also cause seizures, and spreading chest pain.[51] The side effects of Adderall are also similar to the side effects of methylphenidate, however, it may also cause hair loss.[52] According to Dr. Gur Roshwalb, M.D., "There are several possible reasons [as to why individuals taking psychostimulants may experience off target side effects], one might be too high a dose.

---

[50] "Methylphenidate Side Effects in Detail - Drugs.com." *Methylphenidate Side Effects in Detail - Drugs.com.* N.p., n.d. Web. 28 May 2015.
[51] "Dexmethylphenidate Side Effects in Detail - Drugs.com."*Dexmethylphenidate Side Effects in Detail - Drugs.com.* N.p., n.d. Web. 28 May 2015.
[52] "Adderall Side Effects in Detail - Drugs.com."*Adderall Side Effects in Detail - Drugs.com.* N.p., n.d. Web. 28 May 2015.

The more likely reason is that there are a limited number of neurotransmitters—methylphenidate, for example, increases a couple of these neurotransmitters. While the positive effect on one part of the brain is to increase attention, these neurotransmitters are also increased in other areas of the brain and nervous system, like in the stomach (some side effects are stomach pain and loss of appetite), and you get off target side effects."[53] Although these side effects are intense, most of them are tolerable; when individuals with ADHD are experiencing the serious side effects, they should contact their doctor immediately.

    Due to the intense side effects of psychostimulants, some doctors may choose to prescribe non-stimulant ADHD medication for some patients; sometimes non-stimulants are given with stimulants simultaneously. The only Food and Drug Administration (FDA)-approved non stimulant medications for ADHD are atomoxetine, clonidine hydrochloride, and

---

[53] Roshwalb, G., M.D. (2015, May 28th) Personal interview.

guanfacine.[54] Atomoxetine, Strattera,[55] is a specific norepinephrine reuptake inhibitor, meaning it encourages chemical communication between the nerves that use norepinephrine to communicate.[56] Atomoxetine does not directly increase dopamine levels, however, it seems to lead to an an accessory advance in dopamine levels in the prefrontal cortex.[57] Like all non-stimulant medications for ADHD, atomoxetine works over a long period of time, despite taking it daily; within the first two weeks, patients should see small improvements, however, patients will not start experiencing major improvements until four to six weeks.[58] Although researchers are not

---

[54] "Drugs Used to Treat ADHD/ADD: Stimulants, Nonstimulants, and More Types " *WebMD*. WebMD, n.d. Web. 28 May 2015.

[55] Brand name

[56] Araki, A., M. Ikegami, A. Okayama, N. Matsumoto, S. Takahashi, H. Azuma, and M. Takahashi. "Improved prefrontal activity in AD/HD children treated with atomoxetine: a NIRS study." *National Center for Biotechnology Information*. U.S. National Library of Medicine, Jan. 2015. Web. 28 May 2015.

[57] The part of the brain that is behind the eyes, it regulates emotions, and manages impulses.

[58] "Taking Strattera (atomoxetine) for Adult ADHD." *Taking Strattera (atomoxetine) for Adult ADHD*. N.p., n.d. Web. 28 May 2015.

certain as to how clonidine hydrochloride, Kapvay,[59] works on the brain, they believe that it fixes certain neurotransmitter receptors.[60] Kapvay is an alpha-agonist hypotensive agent, meaning it relaxes blood vessels. Guanfacine, Intuniv,[61] also treats high blood pressure and ADHD; it works by encouraging the brain to produce adrenaline.[62] [63] Although this treatment option may take longer to work, many of those who do not take this medication alongside psychostimulants, prefer this course of treatment.

Despite the fact that the majority of people on non-stimulants prefer this to stimulants because of their less intense side effects, non-stimulants, like all other medication, has side effects, some less severe than others. The side effects of atomoxetine, clonidine

---

[59] Brand Name
[60] Belliveau, Jeannette. "ADHD Treatment: Is Clonidine Effective?" *Healthline*. Ed. George Krucik. N.p., n.d. Web. 28 May 2015.
[61] Brand Name
[62] The adrenal glands secrete adrenaline. Adrenaline is secreted when one is stressed or scared, and it increases heart rate, carbohydrate metabolism, breathing rate and prepares muscles for exertion.
[63] Distler, A., W. Kirch, and B. Lüth. "Antihypertensive Effect of Guanfacine: A Double-blind Cross-over Trial Compared with Clonidine." *British Journal of Clinical Pharmacology*. U.S. National Library of Medicine, 1980. Web. 28 May 2015.

hydrochloride, and guanfacine are similar, yet they have their differences. The less serious side effects of atomoxetine are: irritability, dizziness or drowsiness, constipation, dry mouth, itching and rashes, insomnia, menstrual cramping or menstrual inconsistency, and decreased libido; the more dangerous side effects are: allergic reaction, chest pain, arrhythmias, faint feeling, aggression, hallucinations, nausea, pain in the upper abdomen, decreased appetite, dark urine, clay colored stool, decreased or no urination, jaundice, increased blood pressure (migraines, seizures, anxiety, confusion, visual deficits, and tinnitus), and numbness or burning.[64] Furthermore, the side effects of clonidine hydrochloride are: ear pain, constipation, sore throat, runny nose, coughing, sneezing, irritability, fatigue or insomnia, and constipation; the more serious side effects are: allergic reaction, low blood pressure and heart rate, symptoms of withdrawal,[65] nightmares, intense fatigue, and increase in body temperature.[66] Lastly, the less serious

---

[64] "Side Effects of Strattera (Atomoxetine HCl) Drug Center - RxList." *RxList*. N.p., n.d. Web. 28 May 2015.
[65] hypertension, lightheadedness, visual deficits, anxiety, and headaches.
[66] "Possible Side Effects With KAPVAY." *KAPVAY*. N.p., n.d. Web. 28 May 2015.

side effects of guanfacine are:constipation, nausea, abdominal pain, dry mouth, headache, and fatigue or insomnia; however, the more serious and possibly lethal side effects of guanfacine are: allergic reaction, chest pain, faint feeling, dizziness, arrhythmia, trouble breathing, and weakness.[67] If patients are experiencing or is unable to tolerate side effects of the non-stimulants, they should discuss this with their doctors.

Medication is a common yet controversial treatment option because some people believe that ADHD does not exist and others believe that it is unhealthy because it can be addictive or it will change their child's personality. In reality, ADHD medications are only addictive to those who don't need them. In addition, according to Pediatric Neuropsychologist, Laura Tagliareni, "...when prescribed effectively, ADHD medications work quite well soon after taking them. Your child's personality won't change. But his ability to focus and self-regulate will improve. This can make it easier to learn and also to manage social situations. These

---

[67]"Guanfacine (By Mouth)." *National Center for Biotechnology Information*. U.S. National Library of Medicine, n.d. Web. 28 May 2015.

positive changes can help your child build confidence and positive self-esteem...."[68] Furthermore, evidence shows that people with ADHD are more likely to become addicted illegal or prescription narcotic drugs and alcohol because these substances increase the lacking neurotransmitter levels, just like psychostimulants. 25% of alcoholics being treated have ADHD.[69] As a matter of fact, 17% of girls and 47% of boys with ADHD abuse illegal drugs or alcohol.[70] Many say that these drugs make them calmer and more attentive. "That was the case for Beth, 27, a special education teacher in Ft. Wayne, Indiana. In college, she recalls, 'My mind was so out of control, and drinking would make that go away. I didn't drink to get smashed, but to concentrate and get my homework done.' Drink eased other ADHD miseries, too. Says Beth, 'The boredom was

---

[68] Tagliareni, Laura, Ph.D. "Will ADHD Medication Change My Child's Personality?" *Understood.org*. Understood, LLC, 01 Jan. 0001. Web. 27 May 2015.
[69] "ADHD and Substance Abuse: Alcohol and Drugs Connected to ADHD."*WebMD*. WebMD, n.d. Web. 29 May 2015. <http://www.webmd.com/add-adhd/guide/adhd-and-substance-abuse-is-there-a-link>.
[70] Robb, Adelaide, M.D. "ADHD and Substance Use: The Importance of Integrated Treatment." *Nami Beginnings* 11 (2008): 5+. Web. 29 May 2015.

impossible. I could be sitting in an interesting lecture and be totally bored. When I drank, I didn't care that I was bored.'"[71] This type of self medication is self destructive and dangerous. In addition, others may avoid medication because of their side effects, however, those could be managed with other medications such as pain killers and in most cases the off target side effects outweigh the benefits of taking the medication. Although there is controversy over medication, and it does not work for everybody; those seeking treatment should try the medications before criticising it.

---

[71] Sherman, Carl, Ph.D. "Addiction and ADHD Adults." *ADDitude Magazine*. N.p., n.d. Web. 29 May 2015. <http://www.additudemag.com/adhd/article/1868.html>.

Attention Deficit Hyperactivity Disorder | Olivia Roshwalb

Controversy of Indigo Children

There are some controversial labels and treatment options for children with ADHD such as "Indigo Children," mainly treated with spiritual psychotherapy, and diet changes, not with psychostimulants and other medication. According to *The Care and Feeding of Indigo Children*, by Doreen Virtue, Ph.D.,[72] and a spiritual doctor of psychology, most Indigo Children are misdiagnosed with ADHD because they are unable abide by the social norms due to the fact that their souls are spiritually superior than others.[73] Furthermore, throughout Dr. Virtue's childhood, the angels, other and other spirits from the supernatural world along with her later interviews with "Indigo Children" and their community have been providing her with information about the supernatural indigo world. For instance, many "Indigo Children" have the ability to "warp time,"

---

[72] She believes that she is a precursor to "Indigo Children," and she also believes that her children are also "Indigo Children."

[73] Virtue, Doreen. *The Care and Feeding of Indigo Children*. Carlsbad, CA: Hay House, 2001. PrVirtue, Doreen. "Indigo Children and the New Age of Peace." *The Care and Feeding of Indigo Children*. Carlsbad, CA: Hay House, 2001. 39-40. Print.

distorting it. According to her "Indigo Child," Chuck, "don't look at the clocks or any other landmarks on your drive to your destination because that will slow you down by locking you into time and space."[74] A main characteristic of "Indigo Children" are their supernatural telepathic abilities, in her book, she writes "virtually every parent, teacher, and health-care professional I've interviewed has said that they notice how 'today's kids [indigo children]' are incredibly psychic."[75] The concept of "Indigo Children" is controversial because modern science opposes the certain aspects of supernatural world.

Those who believe in this idiocy, believe that the concept of "Indigo Children" is real and that some children with ADHD are misdiagnosed as ADHD and not diagnosed as an Indigo Child. Some common characteristics of an "Indigo Child" are: they act as if they are royal and deserving, they do not comply with "absolute authority," meaning discipline without a

---

[74] Virtue, Doreen. *The Care and Feeding of Indigo Children*. Carlsbad, CA: Hay House, 2001. PrVirtue, Doreen. "Indigo Children and the New Age of Peace." *The Care and Feeding of Indigo Children*. Carlsbad, CA: Hay House, 2001. 40. Print.int.
[75] Virtue, Doreen. "Telepathic Indigo Children." *The Care and Feeding of Indigo Children*. Carlsbad, CA: Hay House, 2001. 38-39. Print.

reason or another option, and they resent unspiritual activities. However, there are criteria that need to be followed too such as: constant strong determination, must be born in 1978 or later, stubborn, creative, susceptible to addiction, "an 'old soul,' as if they're 13 going on to 43," psychic and possibly sees angels, auras, fairies and deceased loved ones, lonely (they may retreat mentally or lash out at others) unless they are around other "Indigo Children", independent, desires to fix the world, moody (their moods constantly change from lacking confidence to feelings of eminence), often loses interest, has been misdiagnosed as ADHD, has insomnia and nightmares, has history of depression, looks for meaningful relationships and has a deep connection with plants and animals.[76][77] As a matter of fact many

---

[76] Virtue, Doreen. "Telepathic Indigo Children." *The Care and Feeding of Indigo Children*. Carlsbad, CA: Hay House, 2001. 19-20. Print.

[77] The angels along with other "Indigo Children" have informed Doreen Virtue of the ancient roots of "Indigo Children." According to Dr. Virtue, ancient precursors to "Indigos" originated in a bygone land called "Lemuria" (Apparently, the Hawaiian Islands are remnants of Lemuria). Lemuria was virtually a Garden of Eden. Lemurians ate exotic fruits and did not have to fight for their foods, they even spoke telepathically. Their telepathic intuition told them that Lemuria was sinking. Quickly, they traveled to the West

of the criteria listed above are effects of the criteria for ADHD, for example many children with ADHD are visual learners and so are "indigo children." In addition, those who believe in this concept, react to their child's hyperactivity as their child's anger toward the unspiritual world; according to Liesje Sadonius,[78] author of *Holistic Healing for ADHD*, indigo children "may lash out in order to release this disturbing energy from their system."[79] Furthermore, a parent who considered their child to be "Indigo" may define their child's defiant behavior as if he or

---

Coast and settled in the modern areas: Mexico, Canada, and the United States. However, others settled in Hawaii. They became the Native Americans. The Lemurians lost most of their spiritual abilities when the Europeans came and established colonies. The Lemurians adapted to the colonial habits such as eating processed foods, speaking using language rather than telepathy, raising and slaughtering animals inhumanely, and finding spiritual satisfaction in a G-d that is separate from their lives rather than a part of it.

[78] Liesje Sadonius was diagnosed with ADHD, but she does not identify as an "Indigo." However, she believes in the "indigo" concept.

[79] Sadonius, Liesje. "ADHD AND INDIGO CHILDREN, IS THERE A LINK?"*Holistic Healing For ADHD*. Holistic Healing for ADHD, n.d. Web. 21 May 2015. <http://www.holistic-healing-for-adhd.com/indigo-children-adhd/>.

she dislikes rules because they are rules and "Indigos" disagree with the concept of rules. Due to the lack of knowledge about ADHD, and therefore distress with the diagnoses, some parents look for ways to avoid their child's ADHD label.

Although, those who believe in the "Indigo" concept do not believe that this alternative label is a disorder,[80] most, if not all "Indigo Children," seek many types of spiritual psychotherapies such as angel and prayer therapy along with dream interactions. This includes knowing about the types Judeo-Christian angels,[81] and prayer; these angels will act like middle men between the individual and G-d. The angels also act as spiritual guardians and healers. The *Archangels*, are the angles that appeared to Abraham:[82] Micheal, the angel responsible for self clarity; Raphael, the physical healer; Gabriel helps parents conceive; and Uriel offers emotional guidance. According to Dr. Virtue, the *Ascended Masters* were earth's "great teachers, and now they help humanity from their location in the astral

---

[80] Rather, they believe that "Indigo Children" poses superior souls.
[81] Archangels, ascended masters, guardian angels, and nature angels.
[82] Genesis, Chapter 18

planes."[83] Famous *Ascended Masters* are: Jesus, believed to be the healer and problem solver, and Mary, who is believed to help teachers and other people whose' lives revolve around helping children.[84] According to Doreen Virtue, everybody has at least two *Guardian Angels*, and with prayer, people can send more Guardian Angels to others or to themselves. The *Nature Angels*, also known as *fairies*, protect plant life, animals and other aspects of nature.[85] Furthermore, "Indigo Children" and their parents can pray to these angels; Doreen Virtue wrote a list of prayers that one can say. Some prayers are but are not limited to: a "prayer to heal problems with teachers,"[86] a prayer to heal psychic attacks[87], and a

---

[83] Virtue, Doreen. "Telepathic Indigo Children." *The Care and Feeding of Indigo Children*. Carlsbad, CA: Hay House, 2001. 66-67. Print.
[84] Virtue, Doreen. "Telepathic Indigo Children." *The Care and Feeding of Indigo Children*. Carlsbad, CA: Hay House, 2001. 66-67. Print.

[85] Virtue, Doreen. "Telepathic Indigo Children." *The Care and Feeding of Indigo Children*. Carlsbad, CA: Hay House, 2001. 66-67. Print.
[86] Virtue, Doreen. "Telepathic Indigo Children." *The Care and Feeding of Indigo Children*. Carlsbad, CA: Hay House, 2001. 85. Print.

prayer to protect "Indigo Children" from the angels.[88] In addition to prayer and angel therapy, parents can hijack their "Indigo Child's" dream, so to speak. Doreen Virtue writes, "Before you go to sleep.....Say, 'Tonight, while I'm dreaming, I intend to enter [children's names] dreams and have an interaction with them..."[89] Furthermore, she explains that when the parent and the child wakes up, they will have shared a dream, even if they both do not remember doing so. Parents can also speak to their "Indigo Child" as their child experiences REM sleep.[90] These types of spiritual psychotherapies work for "Indigo Children" because they help these individuals connect with their believed intuition.

    Aside from spiritual psychotherapies, "Indigo Children" are also managed with a proper diet. Many

---

[87] Virtue, Doreen. "Telepathic Indigo Children." *The Care and Feeding of Indigo Children*. Carlsbad, CA: Hay House, 2001. 75-78. Print.

[88] Virtue, Doreen. "Telepathic Indigo Children." *The Care and Feeding of Indigo Children*. Carlsbad, CA: Hay House, 2001. 75. Print.

[89] Virtue, Doreen. "Telepathic Indigo Children." *The Care and Feeding of Indigo Children*. Carlsbad, CA: Hay House, 2001. 90-91. Print.

[90] Rapid Eye Movement (REM) sleep is when people do most of their affective dreaming. The eyes move rapidly during this stage in the sleeping cycle.

experts who believe in the "Indigo Children" phenomenon, agree that diet helps manage these children and may also reveal their feelings. As a matter of fact, studies show that dietary changes may be beneficial to those with ADHD,[91] however, experts in this field such as Doreen Virtue, take this to a whole other level. According to Dr. Virtue, cooking, steaming, freezing, microwaving, canning, and freeze drying foods will not only remove the "life force" in the food, it will also kill the "life force" in "Indigo Children." The "life force" in blended or juiced fruits and vegetables only remain for twenty minutes.[92] Furthermore, she ties Ayurveda dietetic beliefs[93] with the eating patterns of "Indigo Children."[94] In addition to beliefs about food and the "life force," and Ayurveda, she also explores the meaning of eating certain foods such as: beer,

---

[91] Boris, Marvin, MD, and Francine S. Mandel, PhD. "Foods and Additives Are Common Causes of the Attention Deficit Hyperactive Disorder in Children." *Annals of Allergy* 73 (1994): 462+. Web. 25 May 2015.
[92] Virtue, Doreen. *The Care and Feeding of Indigo Children*. Carlsbad, CA: Hay House, 2001. 146+. Print.
[93] Ayurveda, meaning "life knowledge," is a type of hindu alternative medicine.
[94] Virtue, Doreen. *The Care and Feeding of Indigo Children*. Carlsbad, CA: Hay House, 2001. 159+. Print.

breakfast foods, cheese burgers, sharp cheese, chips, chocolate, coffee, diet and regular cola, ice cream, french fries, and nuts.[95] [96] Although some individuals with ADHD benefit from diet changes, there are no trustworthy sources explaining the "life force" in food or the explanation of eating certain foods.

The "Indigo Children" notion is arguable because there is no authoritative scientific evidence proving their existence and beliefs. Unlike "Indigo Children," science cannot use its imagination to prove the existence of fairies, angels, ghosts and auras. Furthermore, according to popular Judeo-Christian beliefs, angels usually[97] interact with the earth and it's

---

[95] When "Indigo Children" drink beer, they crave more love and attention; when they eat breakfast foods, they are trying to procrastinate, when they indulge in a cheeseburger, she believes that they are "frightened by a sense of inner emptiness...," and fear failure; when snacking on sharp cheese, they are anxious and want validation; when eating chips, they are exhausted; when eating chocolate, they desire romance; when drinking coffee, they are resentful and disappointed; when drinking diet coke, they want to feel empowering, however, when drinking regular coke, they are "combating internal stress;" when enjoying ice cream, they are actually trying to soothe depression; when eating french fries, they are insecure; and when eating nuts, they are stressed out. (Pg. 157-158)

[96] Virtue, Doreen. *The Care and Feeding of Indigo Children*. Carlsbad, CA: Hay House, 2001. 167-168. Print.

[97] Genesis 32:22-31, Genesis 18

people from heaven and not from the earth.[98] Due to the scientific controversy towards this belief, when participating in academic activities, "Indigo Students" should be considered as having ADHD, however, "Indigo Children" may continue to practice their beliefs in their home.

---

[98] Nehemiah 9:6, Psalms 148:1-2, "Jewish Concepts: Angels & Angelology." *Angels & Angelology.* N.p., n.d. Web. 25 May 2015. <http://www.jewishvirtuallibrary.org/jsource/Judaism/angels.html>

Conclusion

Appropriate understanding of ADHD, and coping strategies to motivate individuals with ADHD, increases academic, and social advancement of these individuals because society accepts the disorder and allows specific resources to be put in place. Throughout history, the views of ADHD has changed drastically from believing that children with ADHD are morally compromised, to realizing individuals with ADHD have great potential, and from treating ADHD as a decision to impede success to understanding the importance of encouraging individuals with ADHD to succeed. Despite the contradictory evidence that ADHD is a true disorder, some people still believe that ADHD is a personality choice, and that it does not exist. Although there are still those who are ignorant towards the disorder, society as a whole is improving in its understanding of Attention Deficit Hyperactivity Disorder.

There are many ways that society allows the government and schools to improve the quality of education for students with ADHD. The Board of Education allows students with learning difficulties to have extra time when taking exams. In public schools, children with learning disabilities have an Individualized Education Program (IEP).[99] In addition, many schools have special education programs, providing an ideal learning setting for students with learning and attention difficulties. Furthermore, many students with ADHD seek external academic help as well, such as medication, and tutors. Family encouragement is important as well. Fortunately, society tolerates resources for learning difficulties to be implemented.

 The more society accepted ADHD as a true disorder, the more researchers decided to investigate treatment options. A common treatment option of ADHD is medication; there are healthy and unhealthy ways to medicate such as: medicine prescribed by a doctor and self medication. Prescription medication is used to increase levels of lacking neurotransmitters, and therefore helps individuals with ADHD thrive. Those who do not seek appropriate treatment for ADHD or those who were not formally diagnosed with ADHD look for self destructive methods of

---

[99] "Individualized Education Programs (IEPs)." *KidsHealth - the Web's Most Visited Site about Children's Health.* Ed. Arcy Lyness. The Nemours Foundation, 01 Sept. 2014. Web. 29 May 2015.

increasing the neurotransmitter levels such as: illegal or prescription narcotics, and alcohol. ADHD medication is controversial, however, in reality, the statements opposing medication has been proven wrong.

There are however, controversial and absurd alternative labels for ADHD, such as "Indigo Children." These children are considered to have superior souls; they can also interact using telepathy and communicate with the dead and other angels. They are treated with spiritual psychotherapy, and diet modifications; the purpose of these diets are to preserve the "life force" in foods. This is considered controversial because modern science opposes many beliefs in the "Indigo Child" concept.

Understanding ADHD is very important even if someone thinks that ADHD is non existent or someone has ADHD. With understanding comes acceptance, and acceptance brings the thriving of individuals with the disorder. In addition, parents of children with the disorder must also fully understand ADHD because they are the ones who mold, so to speak, their child's treatment plan. Lastly, clinicians must understand ADHD so they can help others with ADHD, and teach their patients' about ADHD. As a finale point, those with ADHD should not be defined by their disorder, by what is not working, rather, they should be defined by their true talents; in spite of the challenges that ADHD comes with, most children with ADHD tend to be leaders, more creative, and they do not have a problem with standing up for what they believe in.[100]

---

[100] Emery, Kevin Ross. *Managing the Gift: Alternative Approaches for Attention Deficit Disorder.* Portsmouth, NH: LightLines Pub., 2000. Print.

www.ingramcontent.com/pod-product-compliance
Lightning Source LLC
Chambersburg PA
CBHW041204180526
45172CB00006B/1194